The Journey to You

An Egg Donation Story

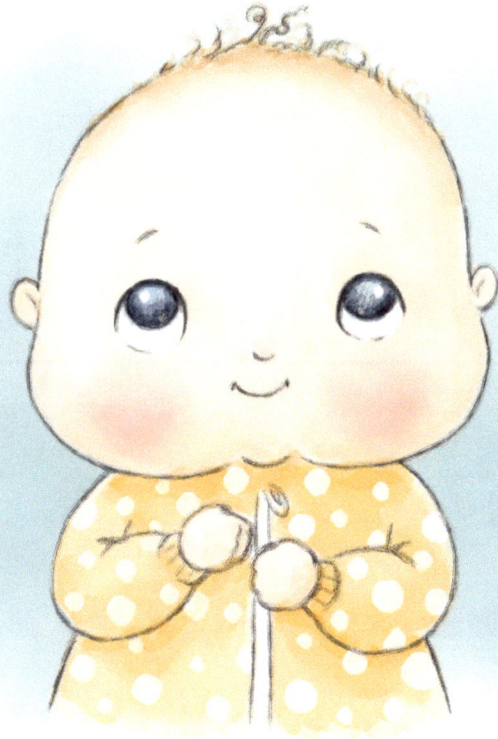

Written by Natalie Hart

Illustrated by Jess Bircham

Let's hear a great story about you and me
and how you've extended our family tree.

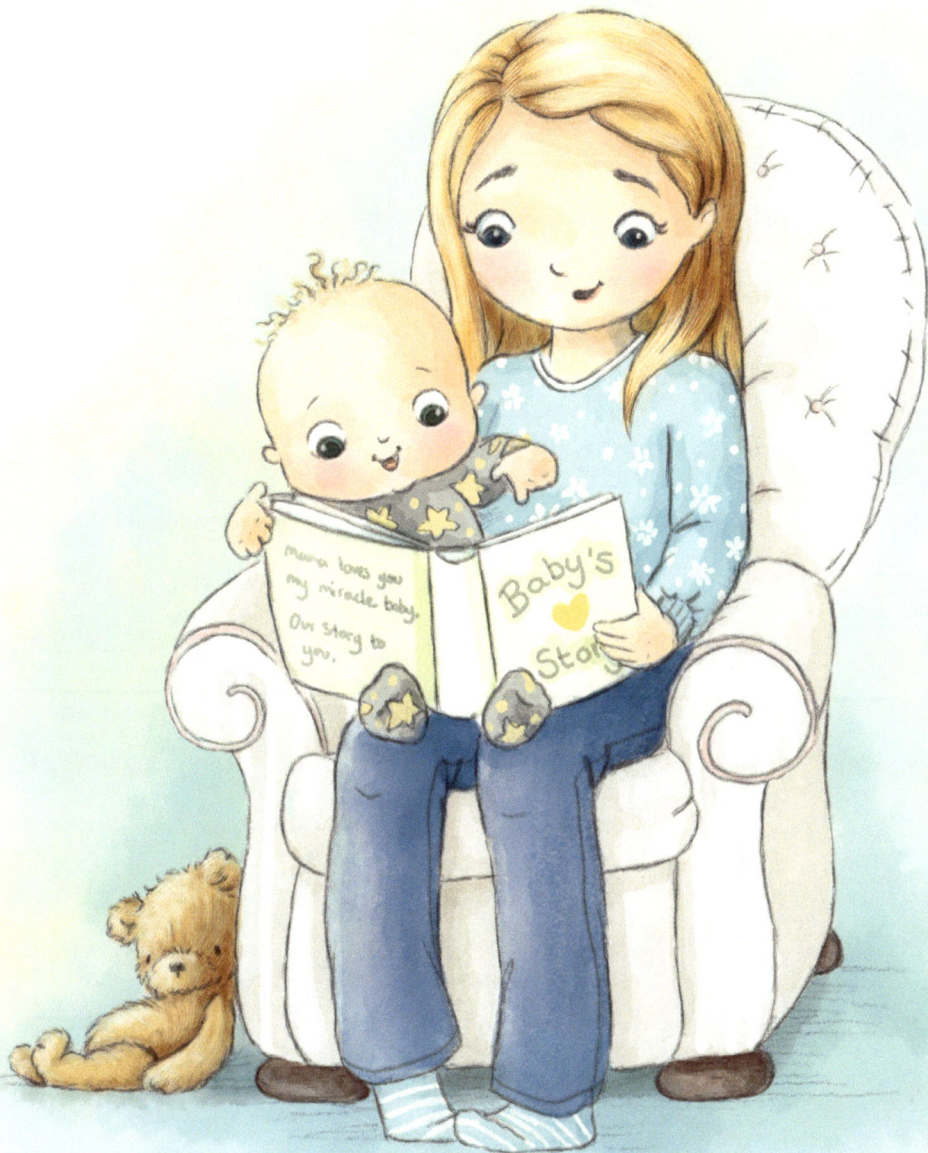

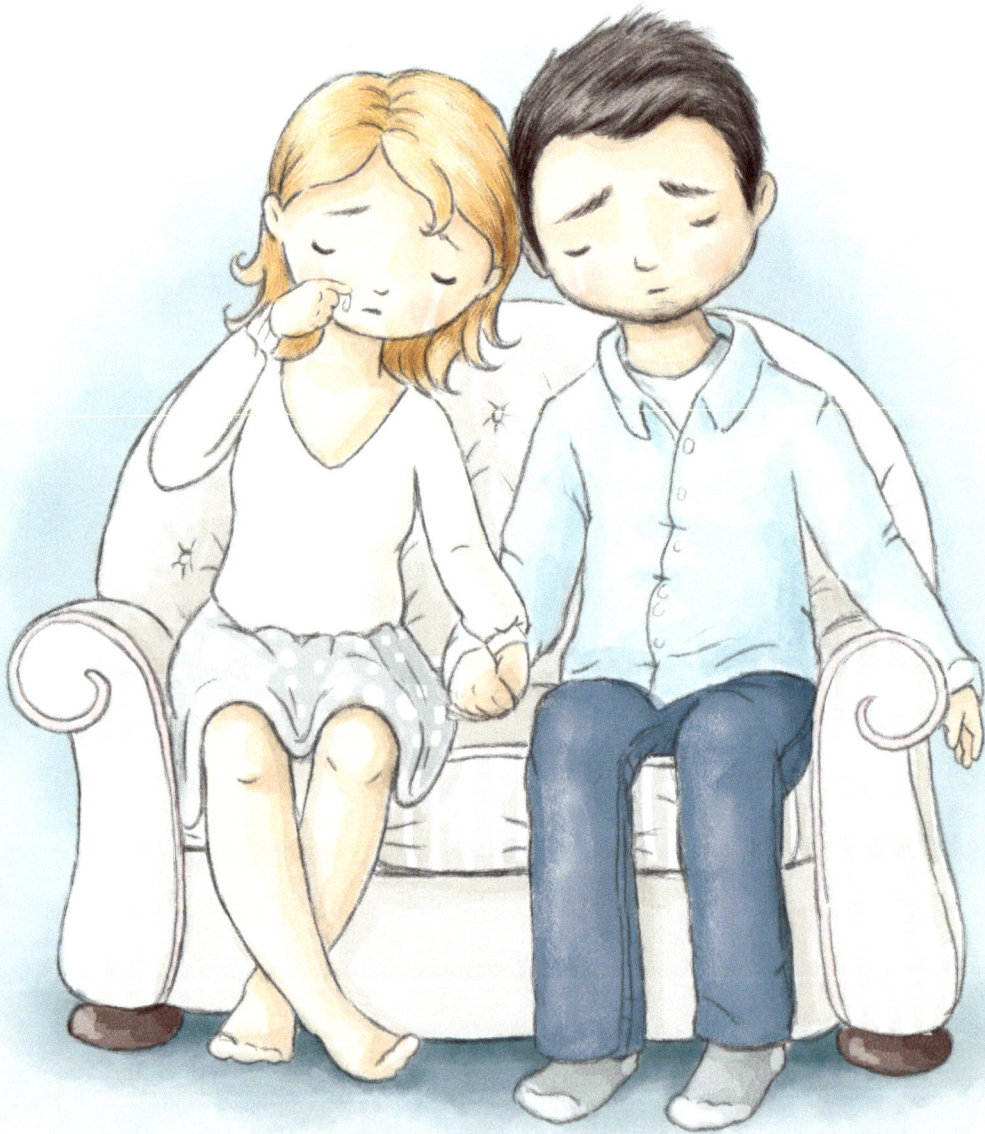

A long time ago, long before you were here,
your Mummy and Daddy shed many a tear.

We both were so happy. But that wasn't all,
as something was missing: a baby so small.

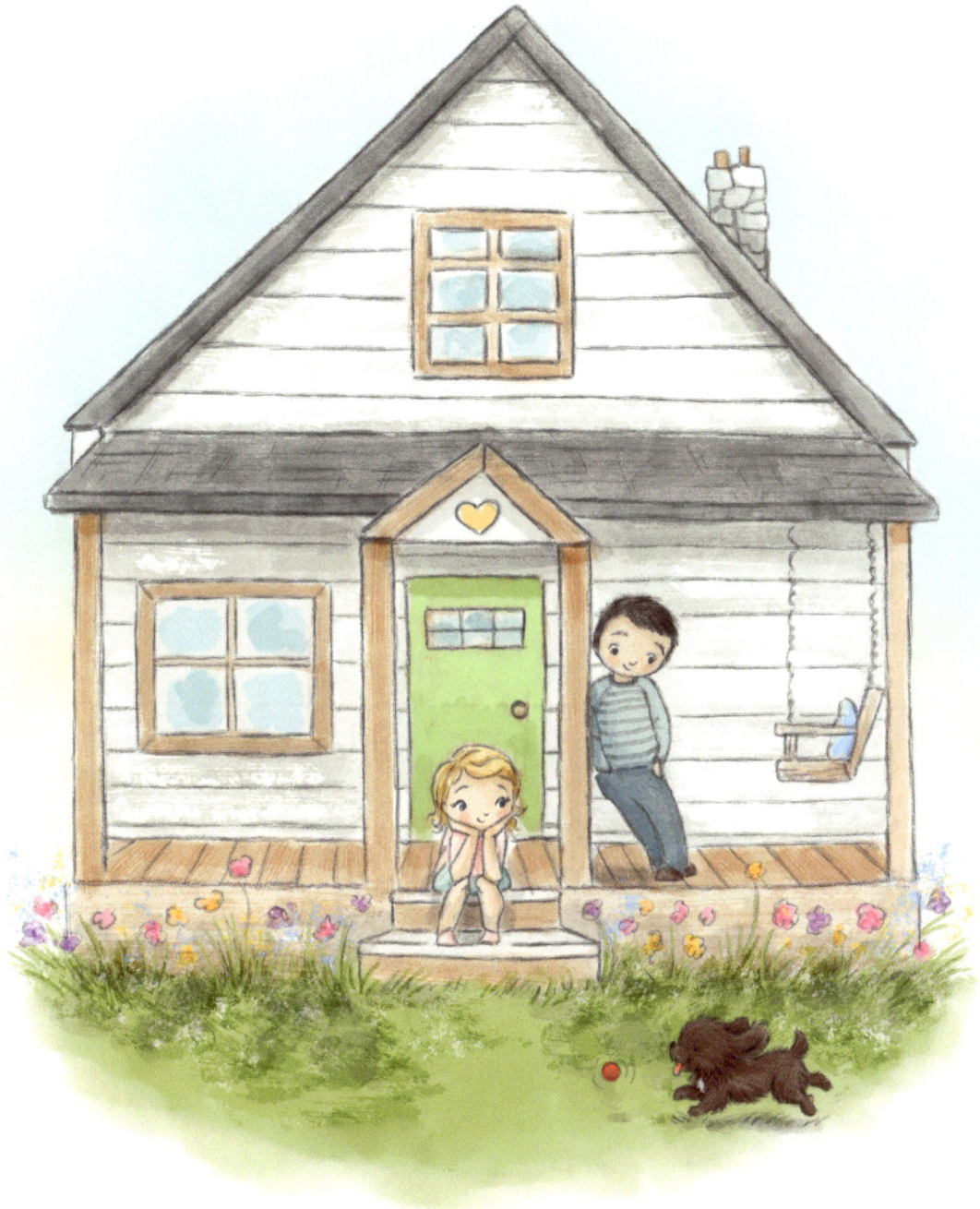

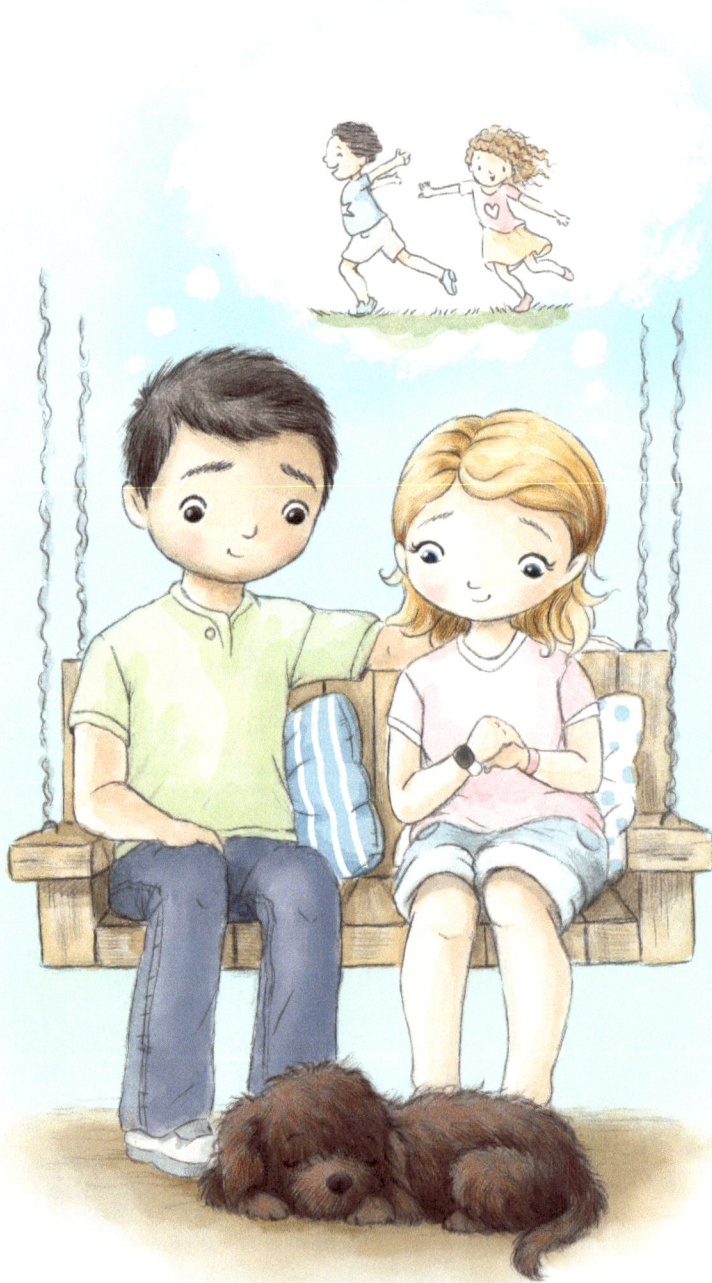

Outside we would sit, and we'd dream of kids roaring.
But all we could hear was our sweet puppy snoring!

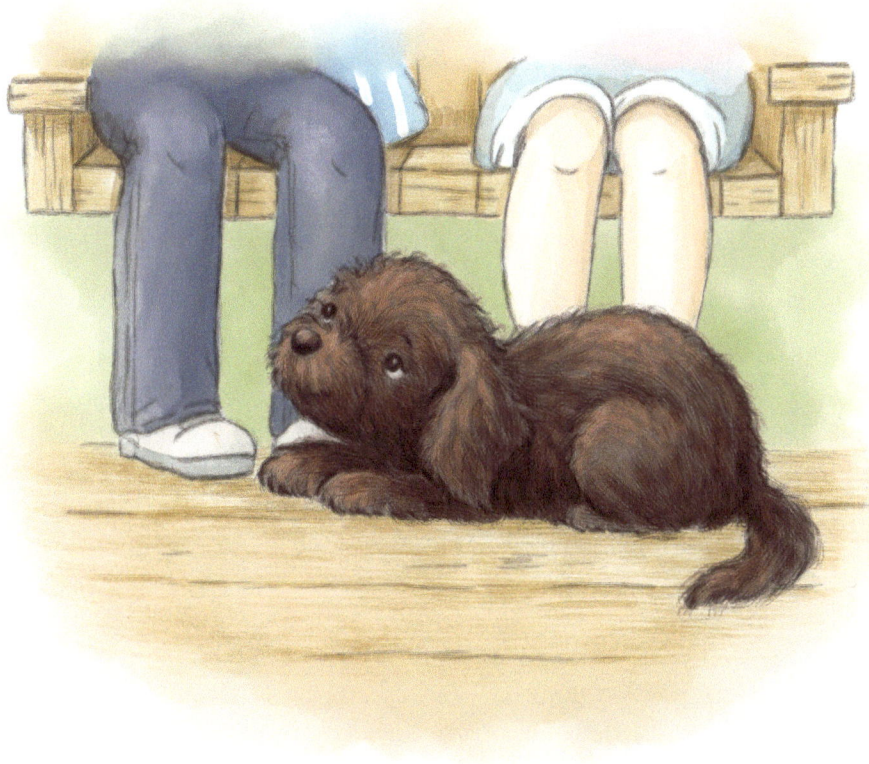

We knew that a baby would make us complete.
But nothing! No pitter and patter of feet.

"What now?" Daddy asked. "Oh, just where should we go?"

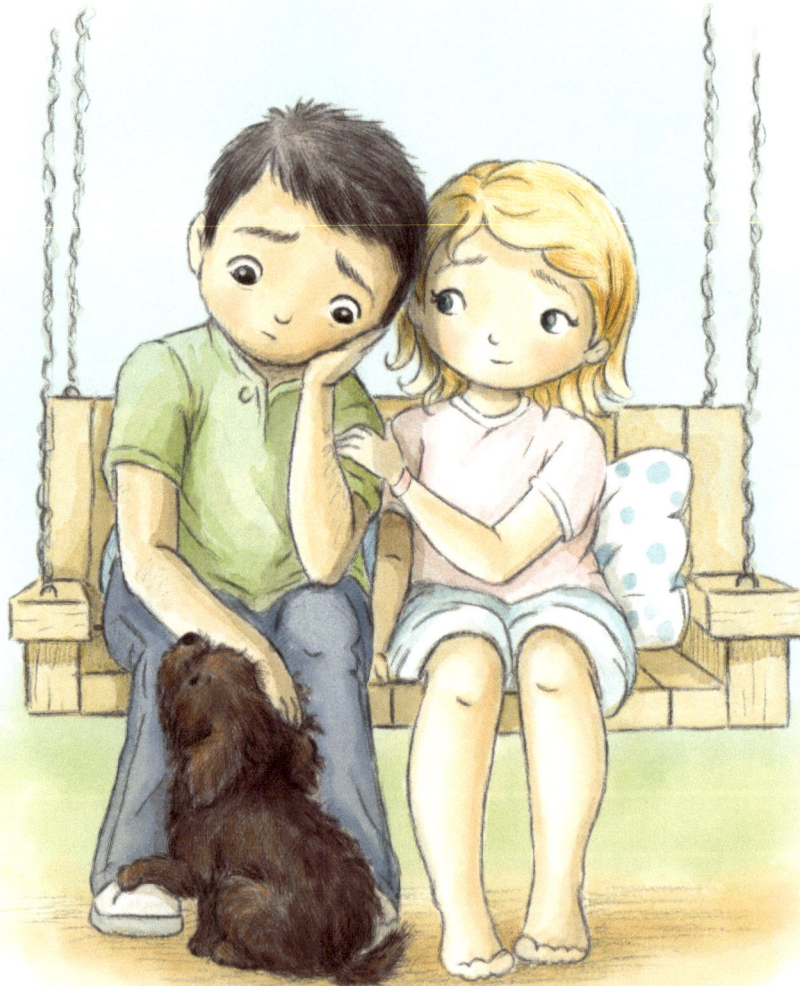

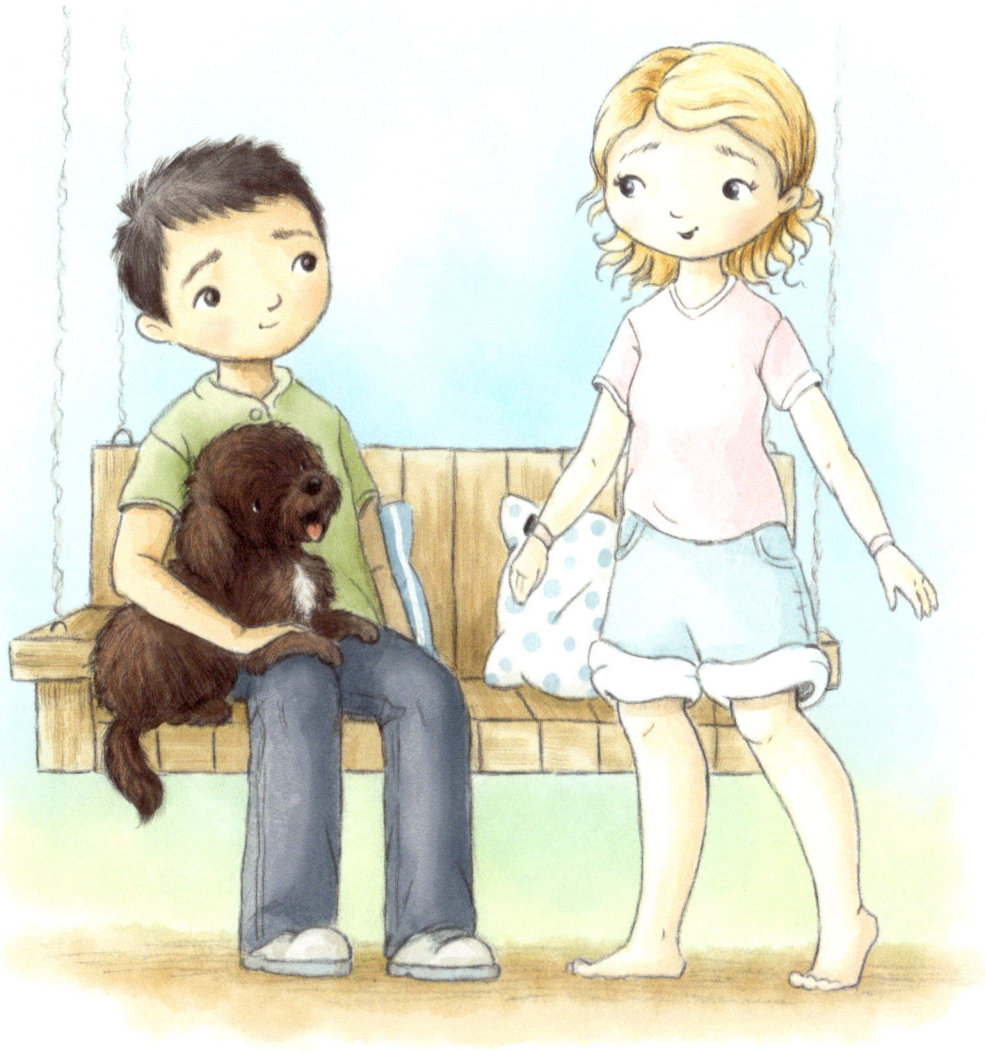

"To the doctor," said Mummy. "I'm sure they will know!"

We went to the doctor and patiently waited
to find out why a baby had not been created.

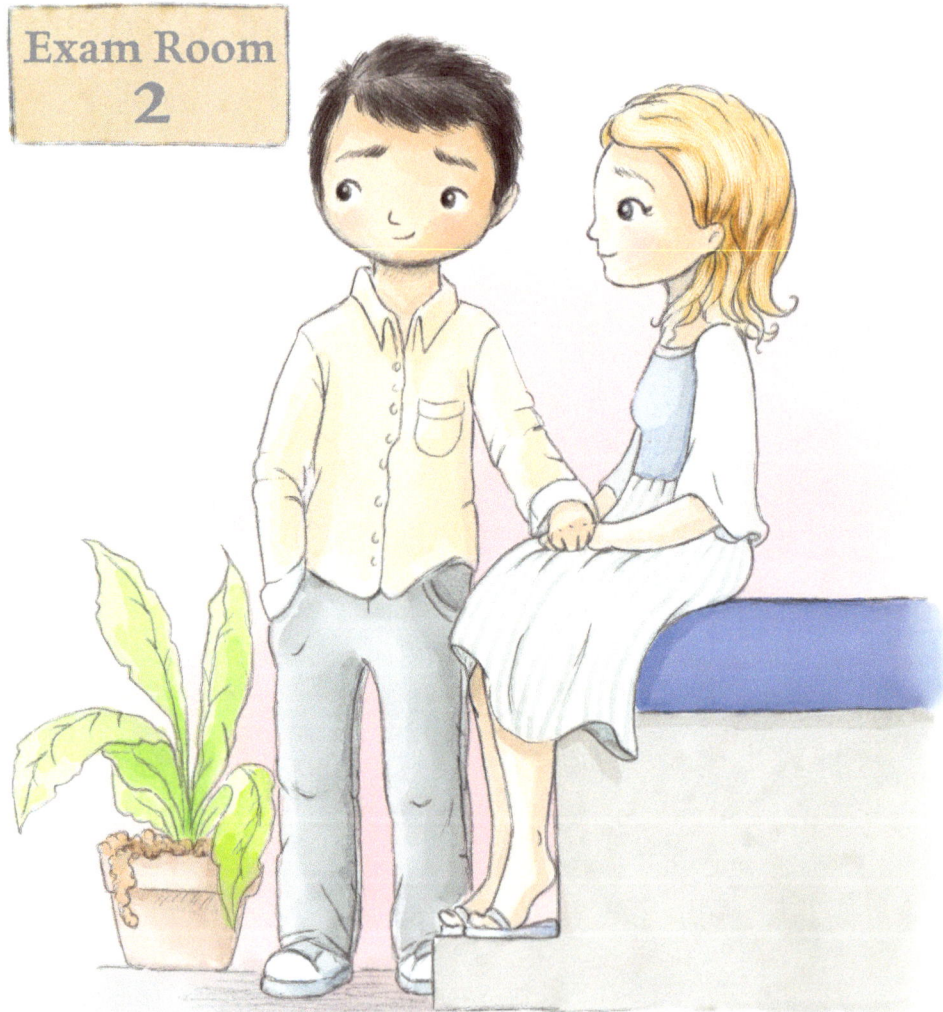

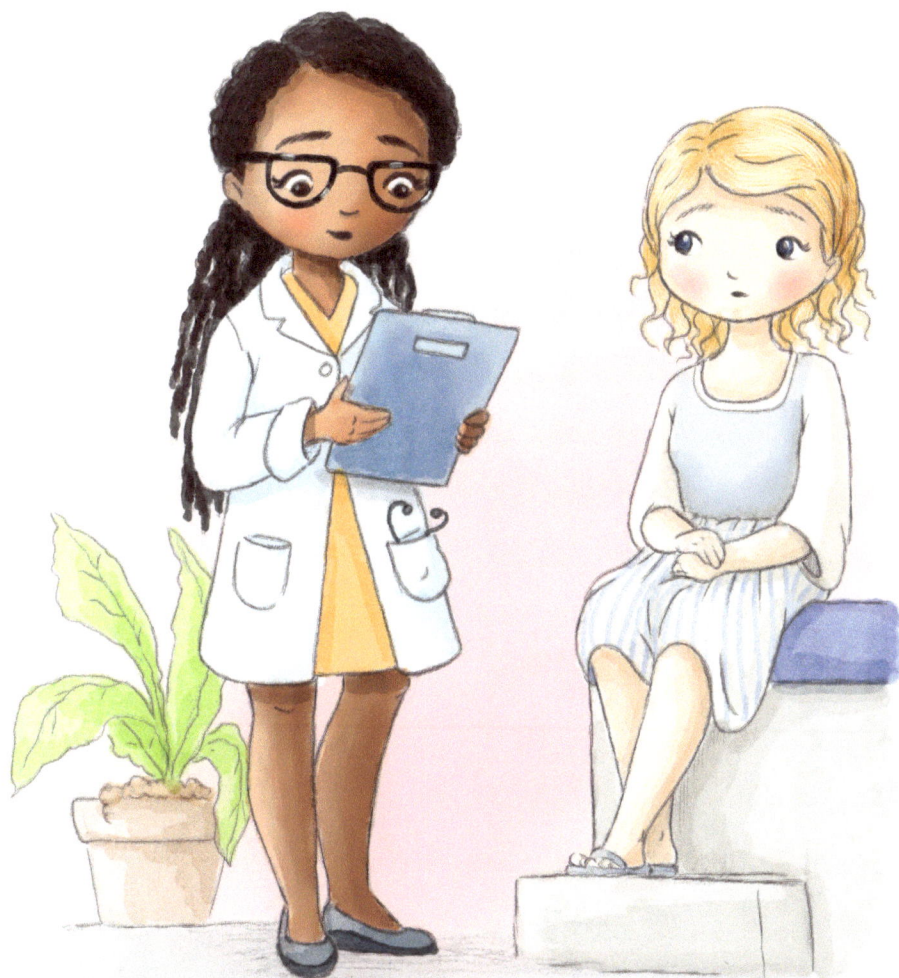

"You need a new egg," said the doc to your Mum.
"So a baby can grow from this egg in your tum."

The doctor then said, "For your dreams to come true, an angel is needed." That's how we'd have **you**!

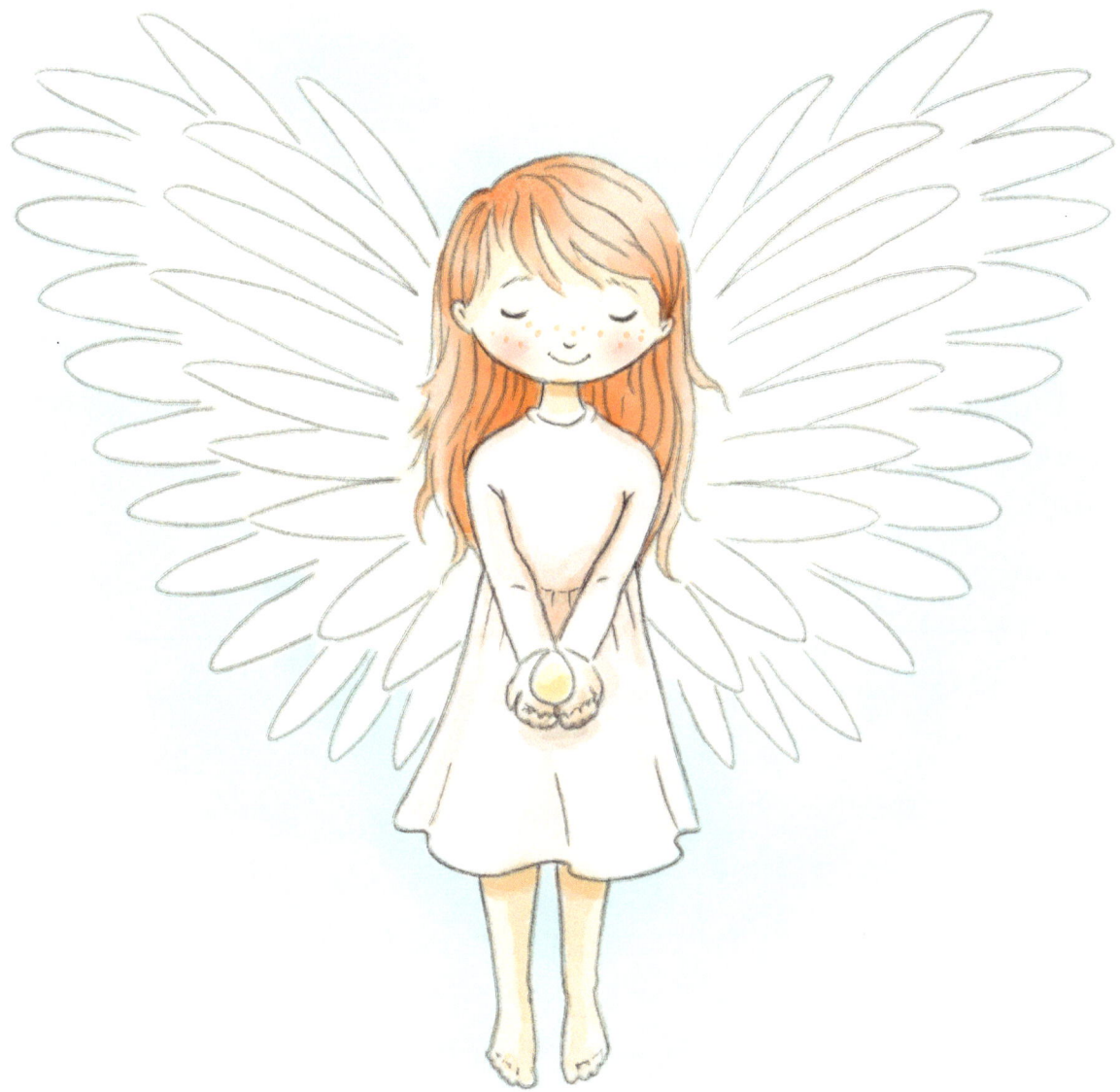

There was one precious egg! But where could it be found?
We searched high and low, and we asked all around.

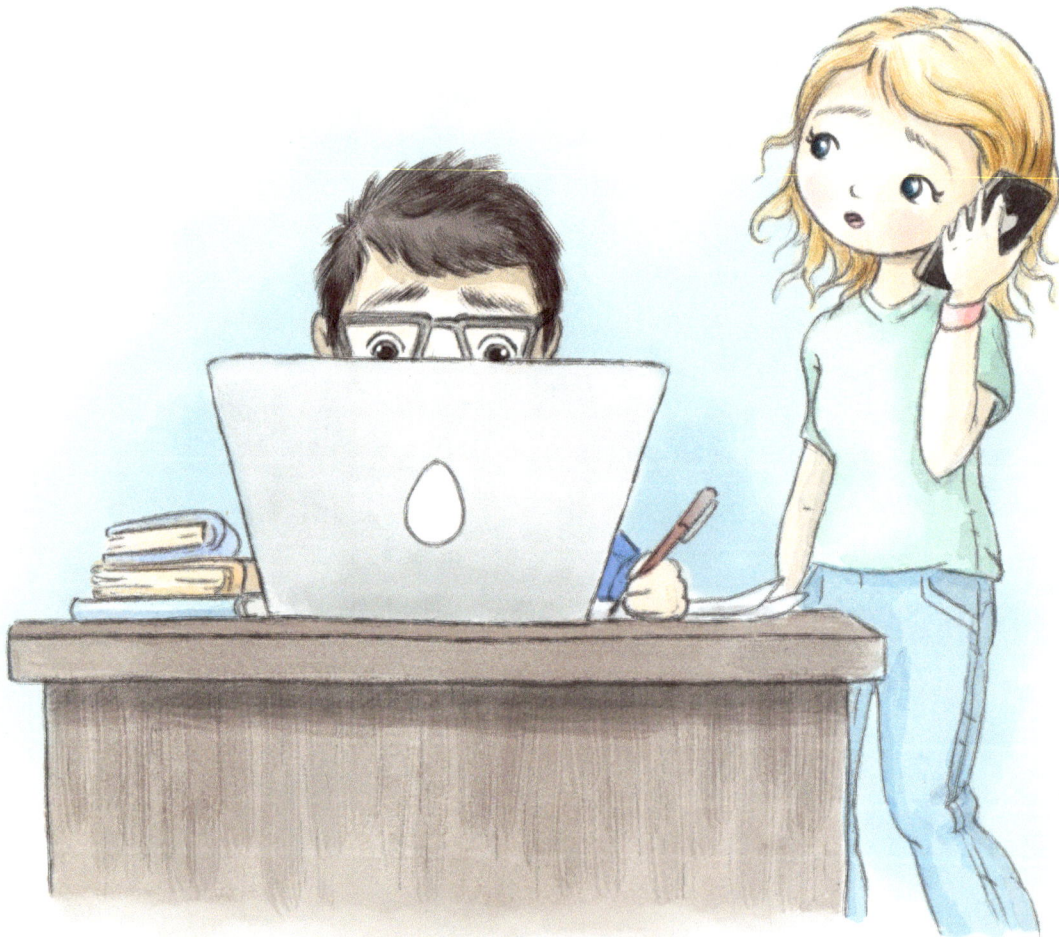

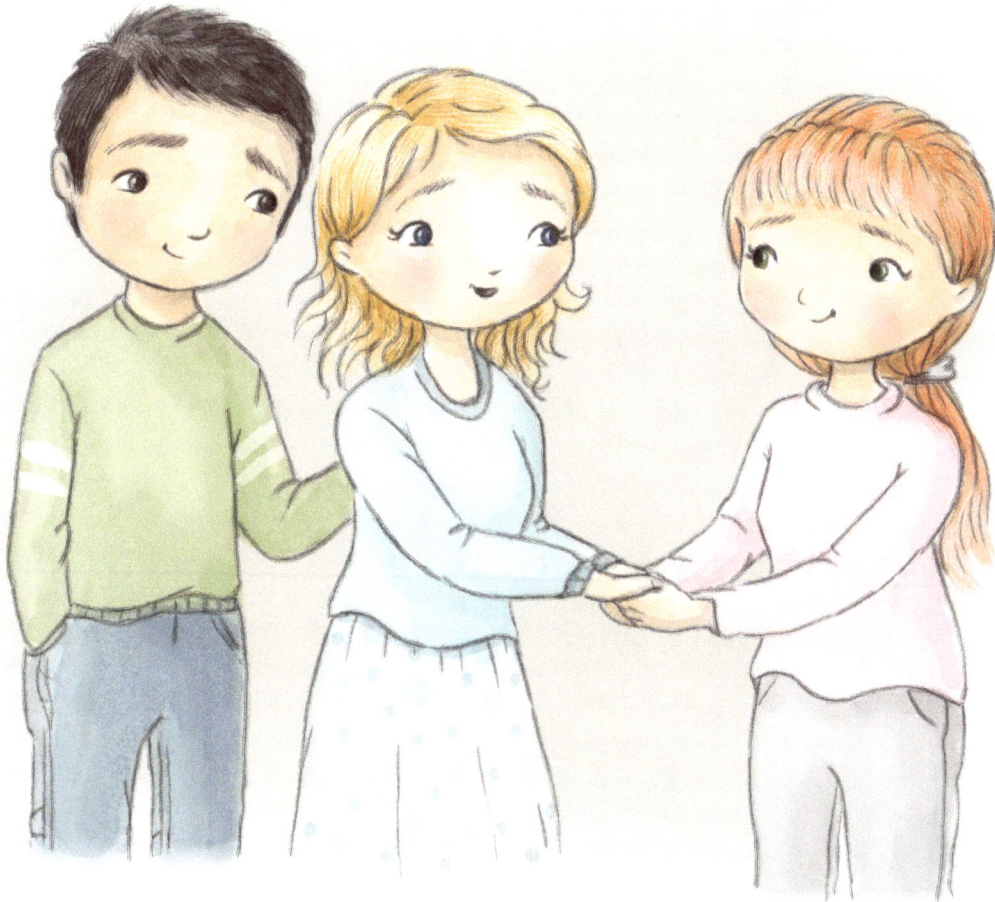

We found a kind lady, an angel, you know,
and **SHE** had the egg that would help you to grow.

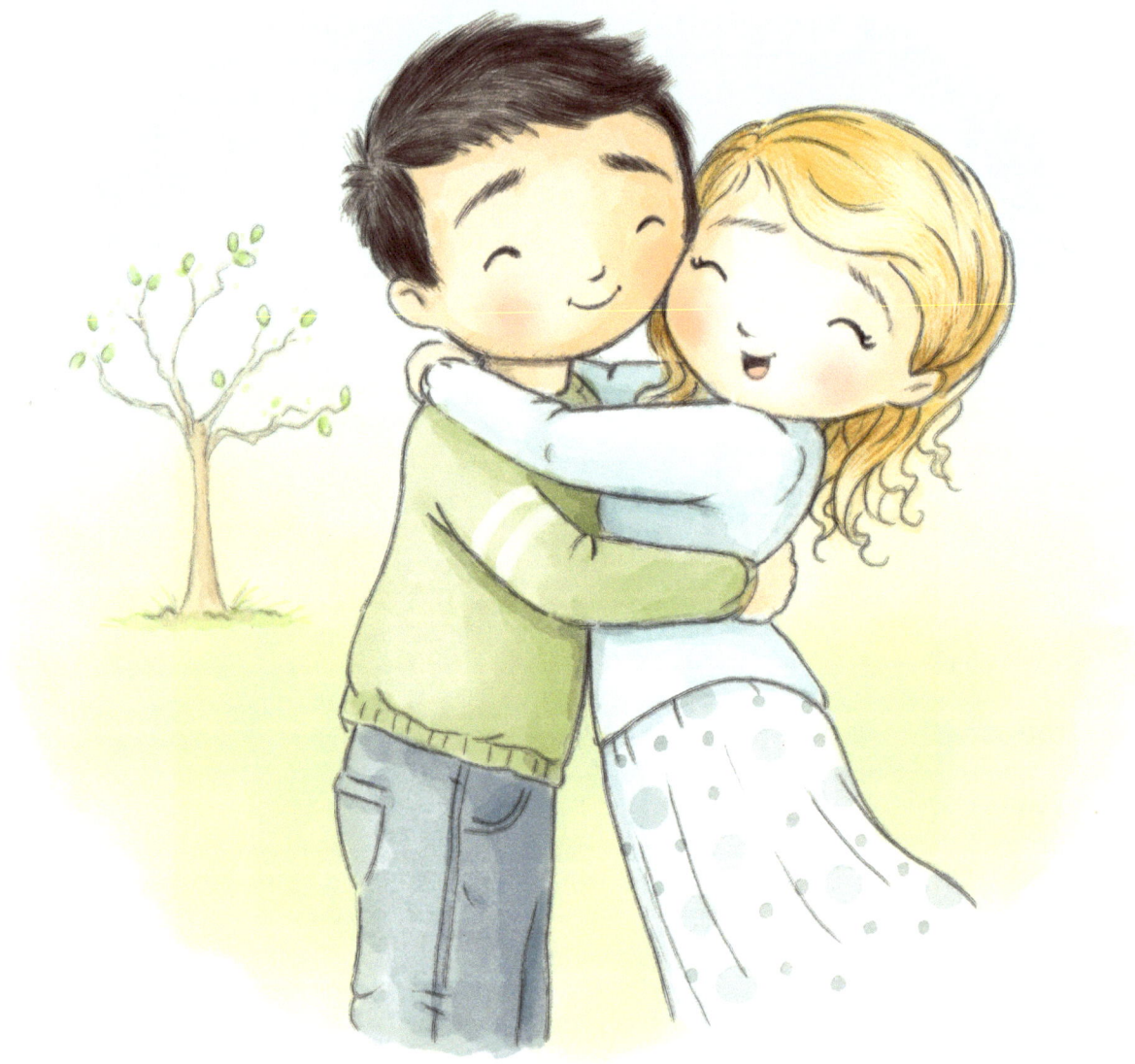

So Mummy and Daddy felt blessed as could be.
Our dreams had come true for our family tree!

We went back to the doc, our best present in tow.
We sat and we waited to see if you'd grow.

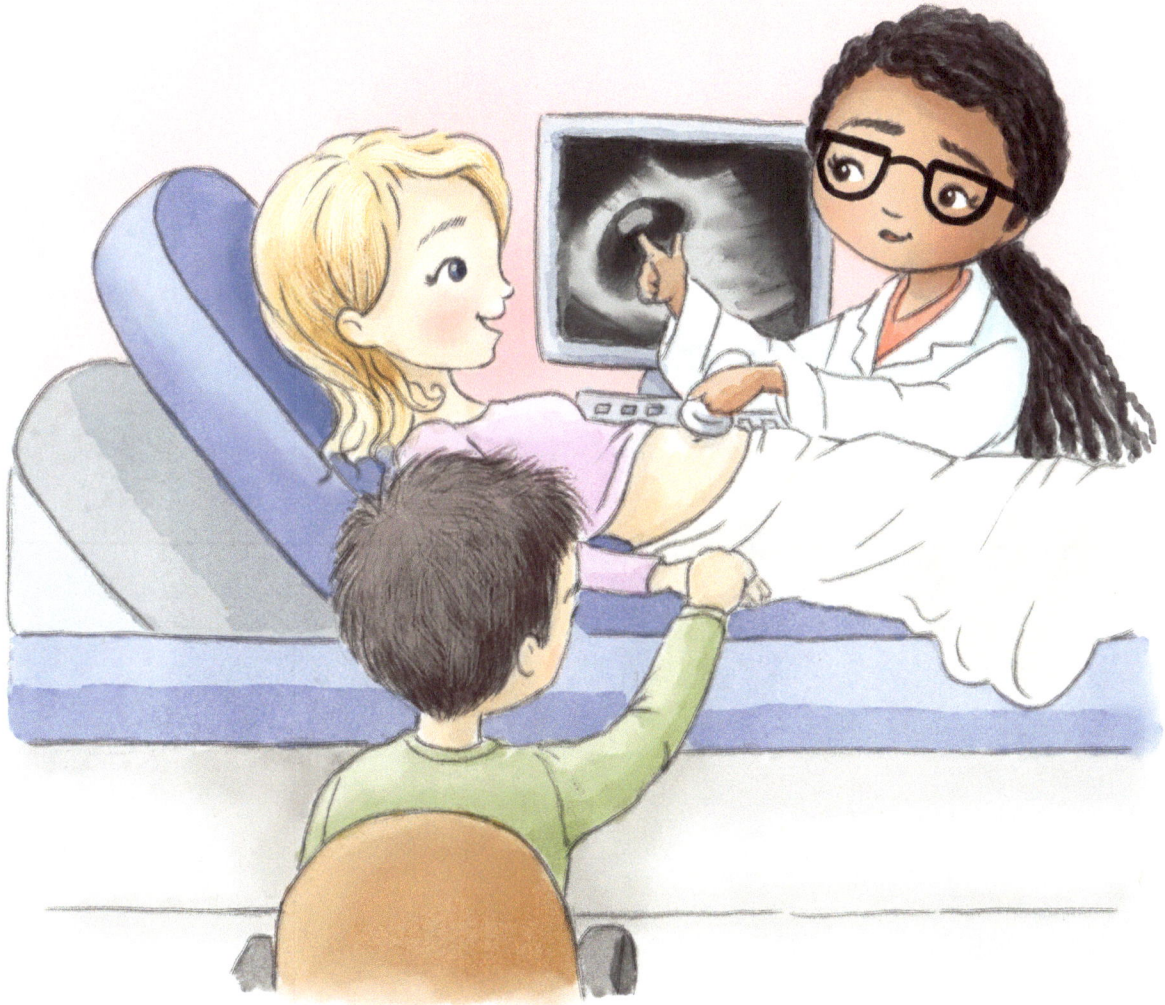

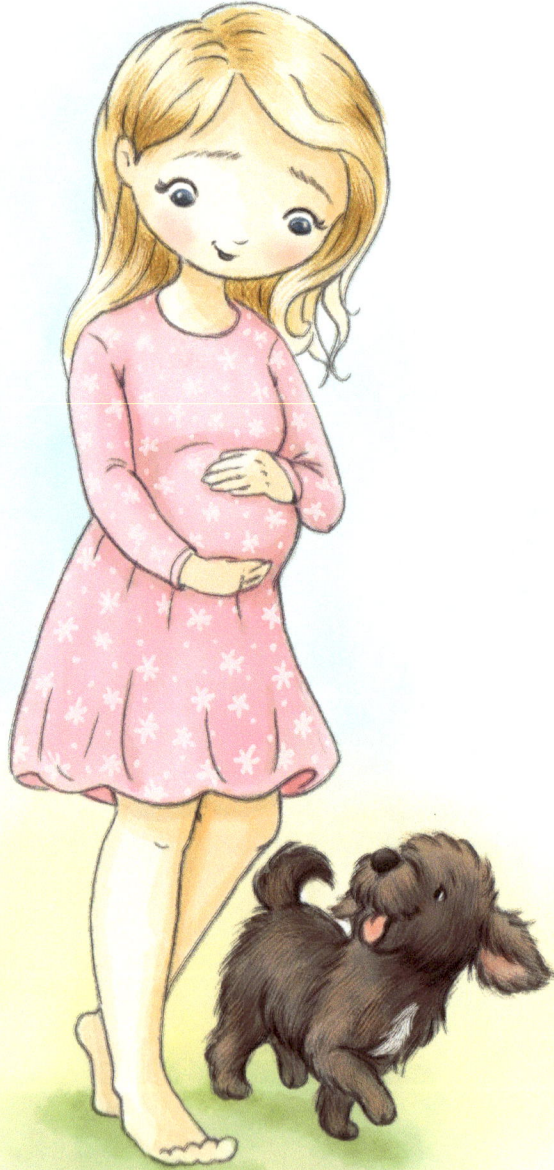

You grew in Mum's tummy. You kicked, and you tickled.
Oh, how you got bigger and how Mummy giggled!

The months quickly passed, and you came to be here.

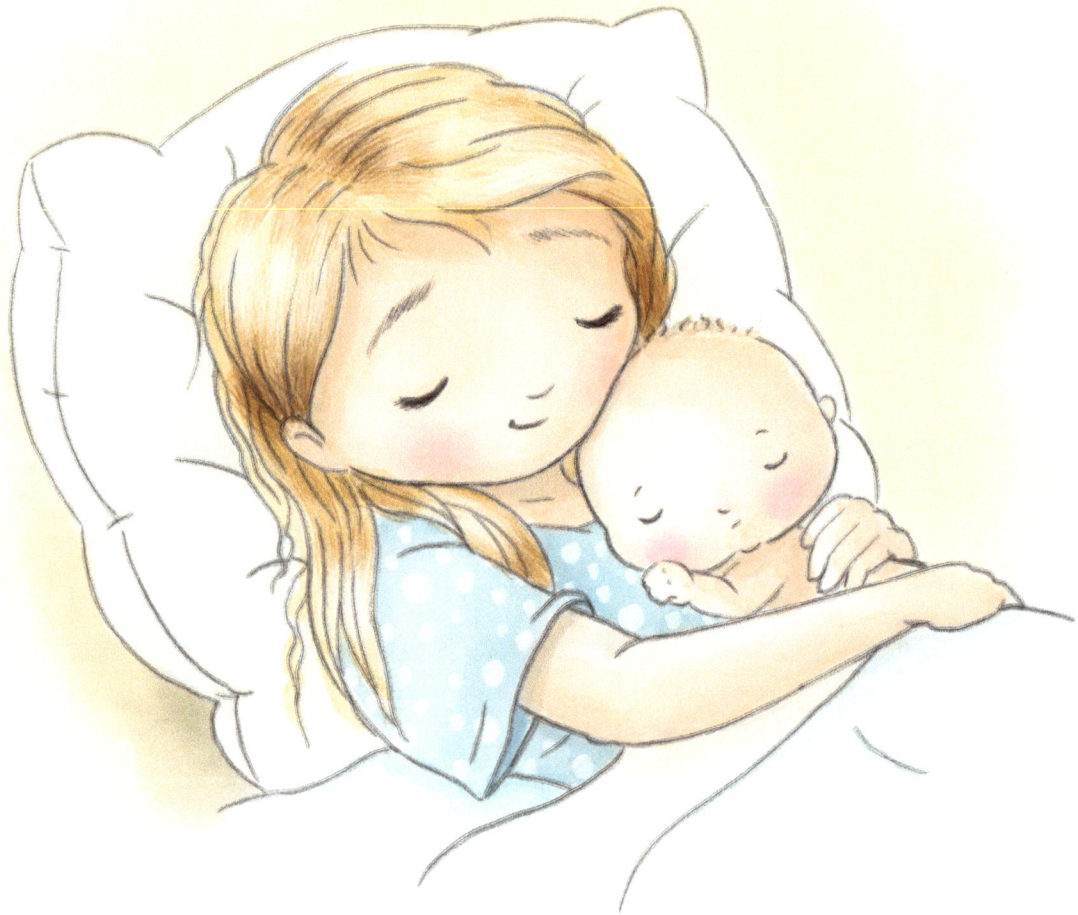

Our friends were excited. They let out a cheer!

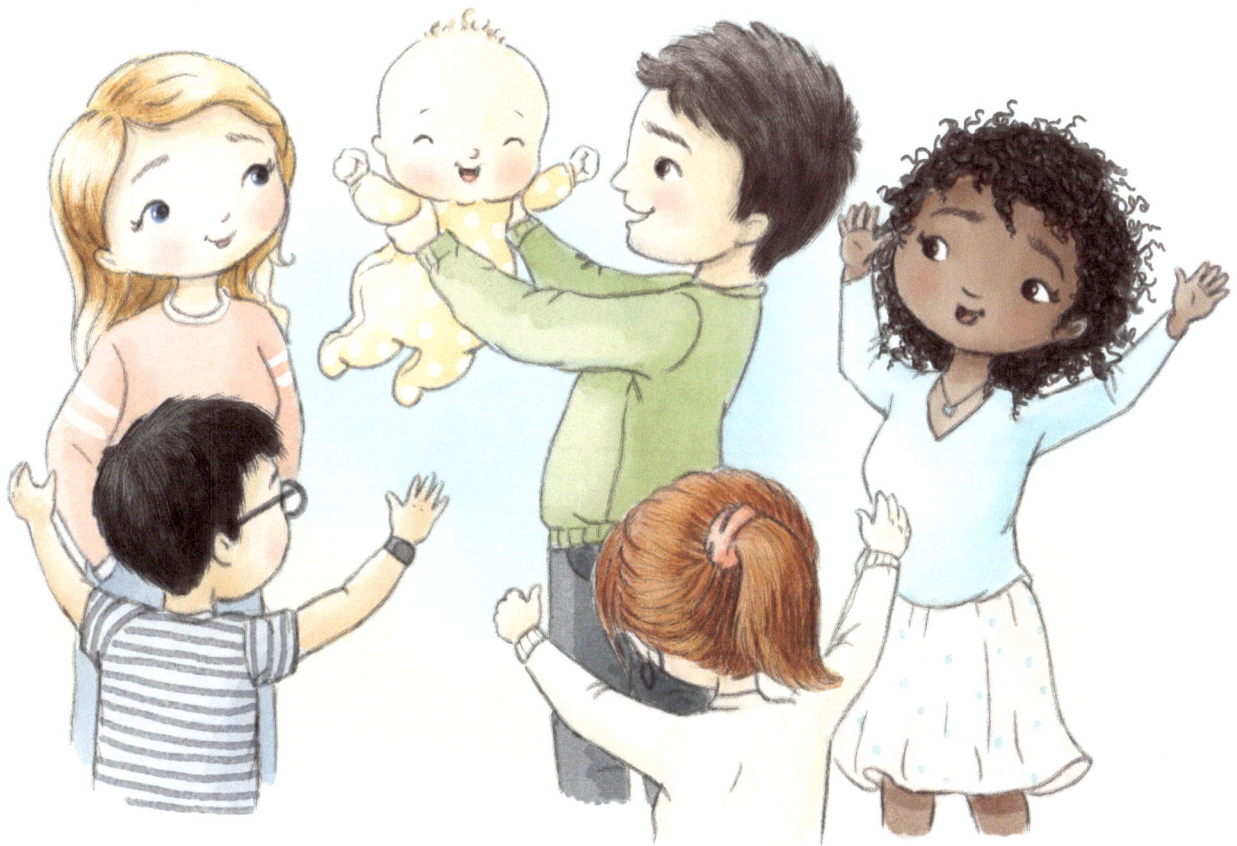

The kind lady's heart made our family complete.
Thanks to her, we have you now, so kind and so sweet.

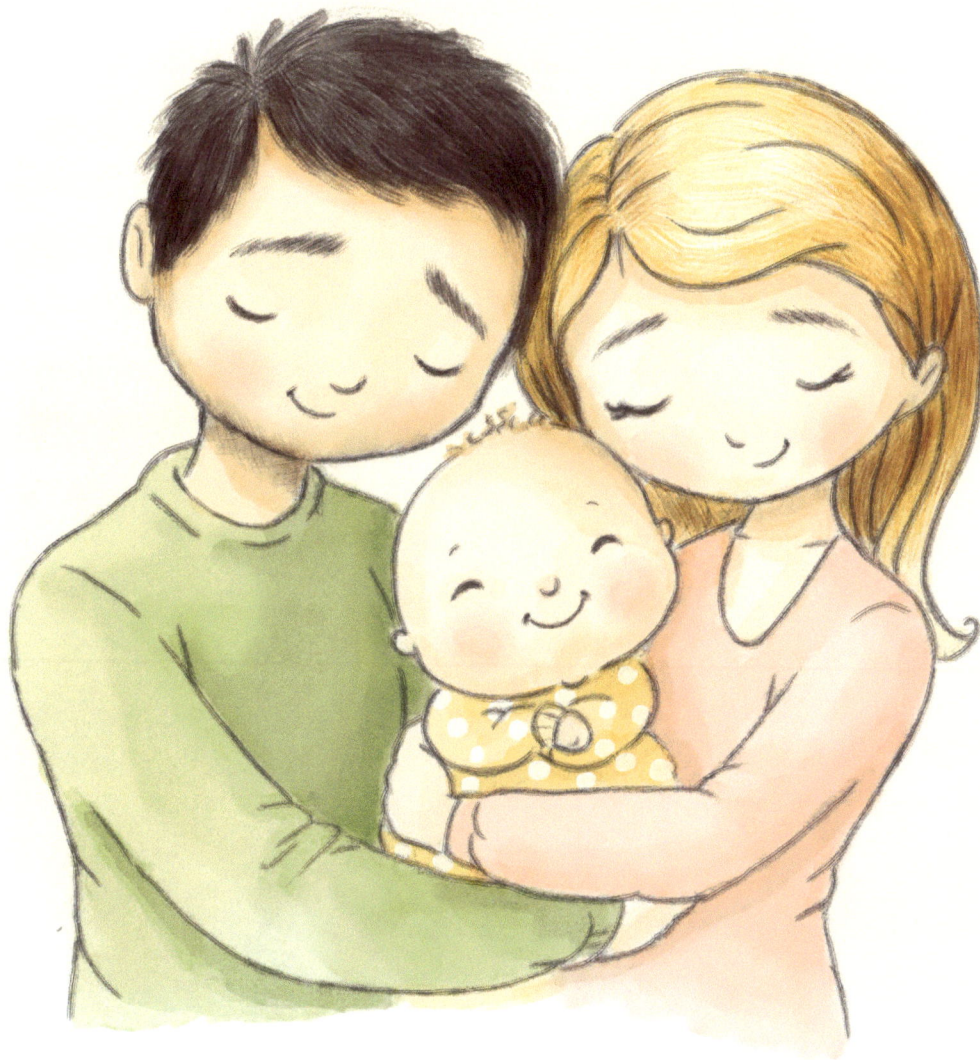

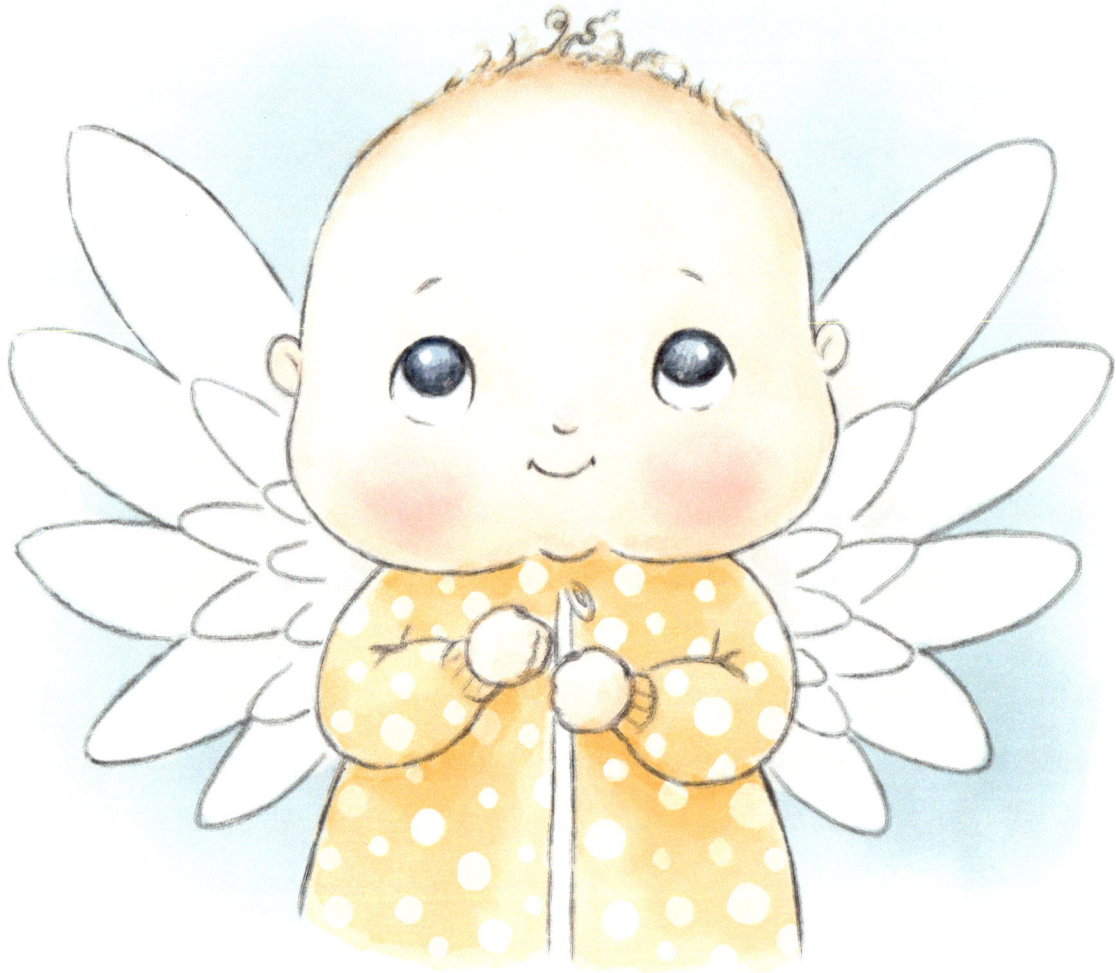

We love you so much, and we're glad you're a part of the angel who helped us. She's still in our hearts.

So, that is the story how you came to be.
You're the most treasured part of our family!

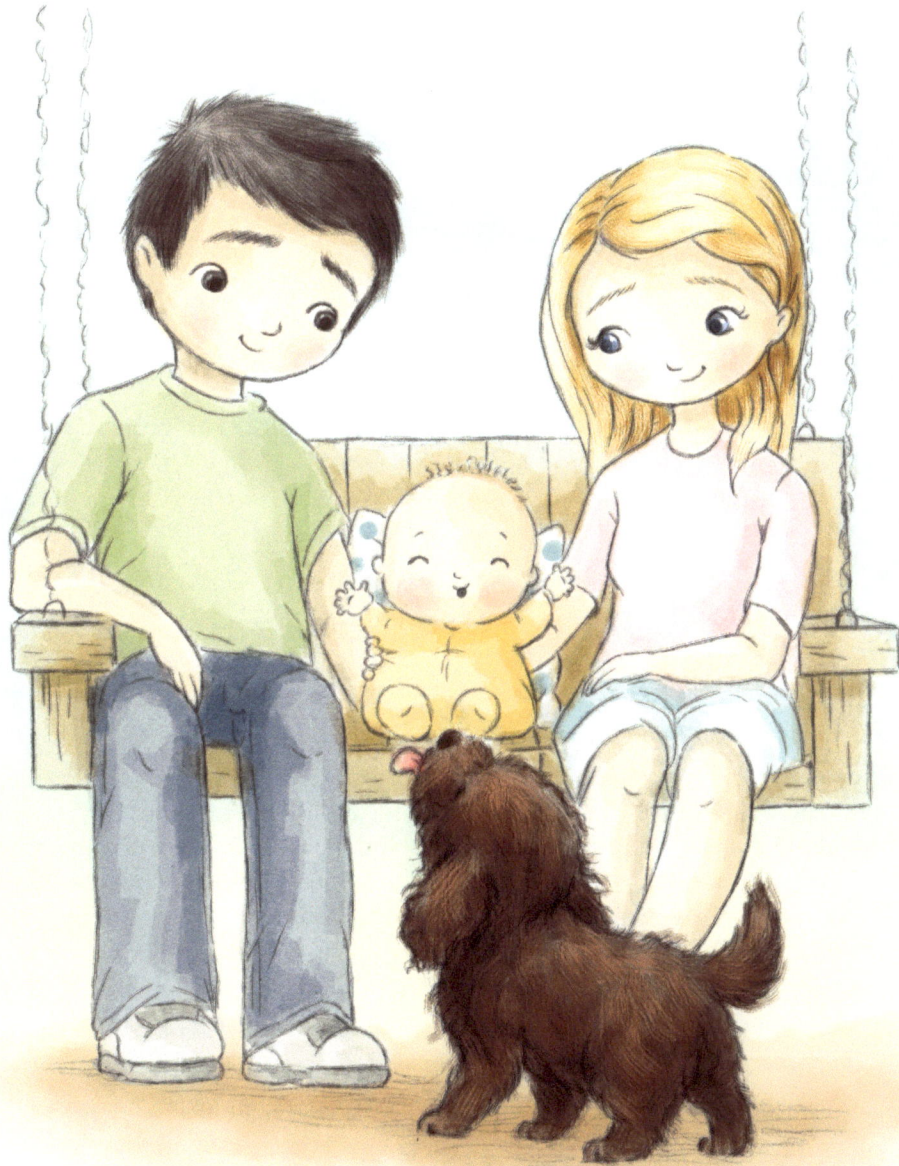

This book is dedicated to my husband, Glenn, who gave me the most beautiful gift: our son, Jenson. Plus a special thank you to the wonderful woman who helped make this happen—I will be eternally grateful.

About the author

Natalie Hart lives in Melbourne, Australia, and is a proud donor egg mum who loves nothing more than sharing her story and supporting others who are about to embark on this amazing journey.

She is passionate about helping families educate their children about how they were conceived. This inspired her debut book, *The Journey to You: An Egg Donation Story*. This story holds a very special place in Natalie's family's hearts, and she hopes the same for your family too!

This book is the first of many other donor conception books Natalie plans to write. Follow her journey on Instagram and Facebook.

 thejourneytoyouchildrensbook

thejourneytoyouchildrensbook.com

About the illustrator

Jess Bircham has been illustrating children's books for the past 10 years. She is most comfortable with a pencil in her hand and a sketchbook full of her fun and whimsical characters.

Jess was raised in Bath, England, and much of her art is inspired by her early years growing up in the English countryside. She is a mother of two incredibly gifted boys and lives in a storybook log cabin in the mountains of Washington State, USA, with her husband, children, horses, dogs, cats and chickens!

Jess has a passion for animals and nature and loves to spend time outdoors and riding her horses.

 jessbirchamillustration

Published in Australia by
DC Media
www.thejourneytoyouchildrensbook.com
natalie@thejourneytoyouchildrensbook.com

First published in Australia in 2021
Copyright © Natalie Hart / The Journey To You Children's Book 2021

ISBN 978-0-6452341-8-3 (paperback)
ISBN 978-0-6452341-9-0 (hardback)
ISBN 978-1-7635364-0-1 (epub)

A catalogue record for this book is available from the National Library of Australia.

Illustrations by Jess Bircham ~ instagram.com/jessbirchamillustration
Graphic design and layout by Tess McCabe ~ tessmccabe.com.au
Printed by Ingram Spark

Disclaimer: All care has been taken in the preparation of the information herein, but no responsibility can be accepted by the publisher or author for any damages resulting from the misinterpretation of this work. All contact details given in this book were current at the time of publication, but are subject to change.

www.ingramcontent.com/pod-product-compliance
Lightning Source LLC
Chambersburg PA
CBHW040932050426

42334CB00049B/81